This notebook belongs to

_____

MY REGIMEN LIST

	Used For	# in Bottle	Dosage

NOTES

MONTHLY SCHEDULE

MONTH _____

MORNING

NIGHT

NOTES

MONTHLY SCHEDULE

MONTH _____

MORNING									

NIGHT									

NOTES

MONTHLY SCHEDULE

MONTH _____

MORNING

NIGHT

NOTES

MONTHLY SCHEDULE

MONTH _____

MORNING

NIGHT

NOTES

MONTHLY SCHEDULE

MONTH _____

MORNING

NIGHT

NOTES

MONTHLY SCHEDULE

MONTH _____

MORNING

NIGHT

NOTES

MONTHLY SCHEDULE

MONTH _____

MORNING

NIGHT

NOTES

MONTHLY SCHEDULE

MONTH _____

MORNING

NIGHT

NOTES

MONTHLY SCHEDULE

MONTH _____

MORNING

NIGHT

NOTES

MONTHLY SCHEDULE

MONTH _____

MORNING

NIGHT

NOTES

MONTHLY SCHEDULE

MONTH _____

MORNING								

NIGHT								

NOTES

MONTHLY SCHEDULE

MONTH _____

MORNING

NIGHT

NOTES

MONTHLY SCHEDULE

MONTH _____

MORNING

NIGHT

NOTES

MONTHLY SCHEDULE

MONTH _____

MORNING									

NIGHT									

NOTES

MONTHLY SCHEDULE

MONTH _____

MORNING

NIGHT

NOTES

MONTHLY SCHEDULE

MONTH _____

MORNING									

NIGHT									

NOTES

MONTHLY SCHEDULE

MONTH _____

MORNING

NIGHT

NOTES

MONTHLY SCHEDULE

MONTH _____

MORNING									

NIGHT									

NOTES

MONTHLY SCHEDULE

MONTH _____

MORNING									

NIGHT									

NOTES

MONTHLY SCHEDULE

MONTH _____

MORNING

NIGHT

NOTES

MONTHLY SCHEDULE

MONTH _____

MORNING

NIGHT

NOTES

MONTHLY SCHEDULE

MONTH _____

MORNING									

NIGHT									

NOTES

MONTHLY SCHEDULE

MONTH _____

MORNING

NIGHT

NOTES

MONTHLY SCHEDULE

MONTH _____

MORNING

NIGHT

NOTES

MONTHLY SCHEDULE

MONTH _____

MORNING

NIGHT

NOTES

MONTHLY SCHEDULE

MONTH _____

MORNING

NIGHT

NOTES

MONTHLY SCHEDULE

MONTH _____

MORNING

NIGHT

NOTES

MONTHLY SCHEDULE

MONTH _____

MORNING

NIGHT

NOTES

MONTHLY SCHEDULE

MONTH _____

MORNING

NIGHT

NOTES

MONTHLY SCHEDULE

MONTH _____

MORNING

NIGHT

NOTES

MONTHLY SCHEDULE

MONTH _____

MORNING

NIGHT

NOTES

MONTHLY SCHEDULE

MONTH _____

MORNING

NIGHT

NOTES

MONTHLY SCHEDULE

MONTH _____

MORNING

NIGHT

NOTES

MONTHLY SCHEDULE

MONTH _____

MORNING

NIGHT

NOTES

MONTHLY SCHEDULE

MONTH _____

MORNING

NIGHT

NOTES

MONTHLY SCHEDULE

MONTH _____

MORNING

NIGHT

NOTES

MONTHLY SCHEDULE

MONTH _____

MORNING

NIGHT

NOTES

MONTHLY SCHEDULE

MONTH _____

MORNING

NIGHT

NOTES

MONTHLY SCHEDULE

MONTH _____

MORNING

NIGHT

NOTES

MONTHLY SCHEDULE

MONTH _____

MORNING

NIGHT

NOTES

MONTHLY SCHEDULE

MONTH _____

MORNING									

NIGHT									

NOTES

MONTHLY SCHEDULE

MONTH _____

MORNING

NIGHT

NOTES

MONTHLY SCHEDULE

MONTH _____

MORNING

NIGHT

NOTES

MONTHLY SCHEDULE

MONTH _____

MORNING

NIGHT

NOTES

MONTHLY SCHEDULE

MONTH _____

MORNING

NIGHT

NOTES

MONTHLY SCHEDULE

MONTH _____

MORNING

NIGHT

NOTES

MONTHLY SCHEDULE

MONTH _____

MORNING							

NIGHT							

NOTES

MONTHLY SCHEDULE

MONTH _____

MORNING

NIGHT

NOTES

MONTHLY SCHEDULE

MONTH _____

MORNING

NIGHT

NOTES

MONTHLY SCHEDULE

MONTH _____

MORNING

NIGHT

NOTES

MONTHLY SCHEDULE

MONTH _____

MORNING

NIGHT

NOTES

MONTHLY SCHEDULE

MONTH _____

MORNING

NIGHT

NOTES

MONTHLY SCHEDULE

MONTH _____

MORNING

NIGHT

NOTES

MONTHLY SCHEDULE

MONTH _____

MORNING

NIGHT

NOTES

www.ingramcontent.com/pod-product-compliance
Lightning Source LLC
Chambersburg PA
CBHW080933170526
45158CB00008B/2268

* 9 781093 795455 *